Table of Contents

Eating one meal a day is a practice that many people swear by to lose weight and improve overall health. The one-meal-per-day diet is also referred to as OMAD.

Although the content and timing of the meal will vary based on personal preference, people following an OMAD diet typically restrict their calorie intake to a single meal or a short window of time.

The potential health benefits of OMAD are primarily related to fasting — restricting calorie intake during a set time period — and calorie restriction in general.

There are many types of intermittent fasting practices and multiple ways to implement OMAD.

Examples include having just one meal and fasting for the rest of the day or having one meal and eating limited amounts of food during fasting periods.

This type of diet creates a calorie deficit, which can lead to weight loss.

Other health benefits related to fasting include the potential to reduce heart disease risk factors, decrease blood sugar, and reduce inflammation (1Trusted Source).

However, compared to other fasting regimens, such as the 16/8 method, which involves 8-hour eating windows and 16-hour fasting windows, eating just one meal per day is one of the most extreme methods of intermittent fasting.

A few popular diets encourage eating one meal per day. For example, when following the Warrior Diet, a person eats a single meal a day, cycling between long periods of fasting with short periods of energy consumption.

Most people following OMAD choose to only consume dinner, although others choose breakfast or lunch as their one meal. Some versions of this eating pattern allow a snack or two in addition to the one meal.

However, some OMAD enthusiasts don't consume anything containing calories during their fasting window and only consume calories during their chosen meal, which typically lasts an hour or so.

BREAKFAST

1. Keto Ham, Cheese & Zucchini Bake

Prep Time: 15 Minutes

Cook Time: 35 Minutes

Servings: 1

Ingredients

- 1 small yellow onion, chopped (70 g/ 2.5 oz)
- 2 cloves garlic, crushed
- 1 tbsp ghee or virgin coconut oil
- 3 large zucchini (650 g/ 1.4 lb), grated + 1 medium zucchini for the topping (150 g/ 5.3 oz)
- 1/4 cup soft goats cheese (60 g/ 2.1 oz)
- small bunch kale, stems removed (65 g/ 2.3 oz)
- 2 tbsp chopped chives
- 3 tbsp chopped parsley
- 1 heaped tbsp Homemade Marinara Sauce (30 g/ 1.1 oz)
- 1/8 tsp sea salt or pink Himalayan salt

- 1/4 tsp cracked black pepper
- 4 medium eggs
- 5 slices Parma ham (75 g/ 2.7 oz)
- 1 cup almond flour (100 g/ 3.5 oz)
- 1 tbsp extra virgin olive oil, plus 1 tsp for greasing

Instructions

1. Preheat the oven to 190 °C/ 375 °F (fan assisted). Grate the zucchini. Place in a new bowl and heat in the microwave for 5 minutes on high. Remove from the microwave and allow to cool. Place the grated zucchini in a muslin cloth and squeeze out the excess water.

2. Peel the shallot and garlic. Dice fine. Keep separate. Heat 1 tablespoon of ghee in a sauce pan on a medium/ low heat. Add the chopped onion and fry for 1-2 minutes. Then add the garlic and cook for a further 30 seconds until soft and translucent. Ensure the heat isn't too high to stop them burning. Once cooked place in a large mixing bowl.Keto Ham, Cheese & Zucchini Breakfast Bake

3. Crack the eggs into a cup and whisk with a fork until combined.

4. Blitz the kale in a food processor until fine or option to dice as finely as possible.

5. Place the cooked zucchini in a mixing bowl and combine with the goats cheese, chives, parsley (keep some for topping), kale, marinara sauce, salt, pepper, eggs and almond flour. Mix well.Keto Ham, Cheese & Zucchini Breakfast Bake

6. Line a medium baking tray with greaseproof paper to prevent sticking (I used 8 x 11 x 1.5 inch/ 20 x 28 x 4 cm baking tray). Coat the top of the greaseproof with a teaspoon of olive oil. Spoon in the keto breakfast bake filling and smooth with a spatula ensuring it fills to the edges.

7. Peel the remaining zucchini using a vegetable peeler to make thin strands about 2 mm thick.

8. Place alternating layers of parma ham and courgette on top of the low carb breakfast slice. I like to place 2 - 3 zucchini strips on top of each other and brush the top with a tablespoon of olive oil.Keto Ham, Cheese & Zucchini Breakfast Bake

9. Bake in the oven for 35 minutes until the top is slightly crisp and the base cooked through. Garnish with fresh parsley and serve. To store, let it cool down and refrigerate for up to 5 days.

Prep Time: 10 Minutes

Cook Time: 15 Minutes

Servings: 1

Ingredients

- 1 medium zucchini (200 g/ 7.1 oz)
- 2 slices bacon (60 g/ 2.1 oz)
- 1/2 small white onion (30 g/ 1.1 oz) or 1 clove garlic
- 1 tbsp ghee or coconut oil
- 1 tbsp freshly chopped parsley or chives
- 1/4 tsp sea salt, or to taste
- 1 large egg, on top (for egg-free top with 1/2 sliced avocado instead)

Instructions

1. Peel and finely chop the onion (or garlic) and slice the bacon.
2. Keto Bacon Zucchini Breakfast Hash

3. Sweat the onion over a medium heat and add the bacon. Stir frequently and cook until lightly browned.Keto Bacon Zucchini Breakfast Hash

4. Meanwhile, dice the zucchini into medium pieces.Keto Bacon Zucchini Breakfast Hash

5. Add the zucchini to the pan and cook for 10-15 minutes. When done, remove from the heat and add chopped parsley.Keto Bacon Zucchini Breakfast Hash

6. Top with a fried egg or avocado. Serve warm! The hash without the egg can be stored in the fridge for up to 4 days. Reheat before serving and top with fried egg.

Prep Time: 15 Minutes

Cook Time: 30 Minutes

Servings: 1

Ingredients

- 3 red, yellow or orange baby peppers or 1 small bell pepper (60 g/ 2.1 oz)
- 1 tsp ghee or extra virgin olive oil
- pinch of sea salt, to taste
- 1 tsp pumpkin seeds
- 1 tsp sunflower seeds
- 1 tsp flax seeds
- 1 tbsp butter, ghee or extra virgin olive oil (15 ml)
- 3/4 cup shredded kale or spinach (38 g/ 1.3 oz)
- 1/3 cup sliced shiitake or white mushrooms (25 g/ 0.9 oz)
- 3 slices halloumi cheese (50 g/ 1.8 oz)
- 1 tsp ghee or extra virgin olive oil
- 1 tbsp homemade Low-Carb Marinara Sauce (15 ml)
- few basil leaves

Smashed avocado:

- 1/2 small avocado (75 g/ 2.7 oz)
- 1 tsp fresh lime juice
- 1 tsp extra virgin olive oil
- pinch of sea salt and black pepper, to taste
- 1/8 tsp chile flakes

Instructions

1. Preheat the oven to 180 °C/ 355 °F (fan assisted) or 200 °C/ 400 °F (conventional). Place the peppers on a baking tray and drizzle with olive oil and a pinch of salt. Roast in the oven for 25 minutes until soft.
2. Place the seeds on another baking tray and roast in the oven for 4 minutes until golden. Remove from the oven and allow to cool.
3. Note: You can make a large batch of the roasted seeds and keep at room temperature for up to 2 weeks, ready to be used for topping or snacking.
4. Low-Carb Veggie Full English Breakfast Bowl
5. Heat the butter on a medium heat in a non-stick pan, add the mushrooms and cook for 2 minutes. Add the kale and cook for a further 2 minutes. Season with a pinch of salt to taste.

6. Low-Carb Veggie Full English Breakfast Bowl

7. Fry the halloumi in 1 tsp of ghee or olive oil over a medium-low heat for about 2 minutes per side, or until golden.

8. Once the peppers are cooked, allow to cool slightly. Remove the stalks and scoop out the seeds.

9. Smash the avocado with a fork and mix with the olive oil, salt, pepper, lime and chile flakes.

10. Low-Carb Veggie Full English Breakfast Bowl

11. Place the kale and mushrooms in your bowl, along with the seeds, peppers, halloumi and top with smashed avocado, marinara sauce and fresh basil.

12. Low-Carb Veggie Full English Breakfast Bowl

13. 8 Best served fresh. The cooked vegetables can be stored in a sealed jar in the fridge for up to 3 days and served warm or cold. Halloumi should always be reheated before serving.

Prep Time: 20 Minutes

Cook Time: 45 Minutes

Servings: 1

Ingredients

- 1 lb thick-cut bacon (450 g)
- 2 tbsp reserved bacon grease or ghee (30 ml)
- 1 small turnip, diced (300 g/ 10.6 oz)
- 1 large red onion, thinly sliced (150 g/ 5.3 oz)
- 3 cups spinach (90 g/ 3.2 oz)
- 12 large eggs
- 1/3 cup whole milk (80 ml/ 2.7 fl oz)
- 1 tsp sea salt
- 1 tsp garlic powder
- 1/2 tsp black pepper
- 1/2 cup shredded cheddar cheese (57 g/ 2 oz)

Optional:

- ground cumin and chile powder to taste

Instructions

1. Preheat the oven to 200 °C/ 400 °F (conventional), or 180 °C/ 355 °F (fan assisted). Cut the bacon into 2-inch (5 cm) pieces and arrange on a parchment lined baking sheet. Bake for 15 minutes until crisp, ant then remove from the oven. You can use the bacon grease for greasing the pan in the next step.Keto Mexican Breakfast Casserole

2. Heat the reserved bacon grease in a medium pan over medium high heat. Add in the turnip and onion, cook until soft about 5-7 minutes.

3. Keto Mexican Breakfast Casserole

4. Transfer to a 9 x 13 inch (23 x 33 cm) baking dish. Top the turnip and onion with the spinach.Keto Mexican Breakfast Casserole

5. Whisk together the eggs, milk, and spices. Optionally, you can add ground cumin and chile powder to taste for more flavor. Pour over the spinach.Keto Mexican Breakfast Casserole

6. Sprinkle the cheese across the top then arrange the bacon in a single layer across the top of the casserole.Keto Mexican Breakfast Casserole

7. Transfer to the oven and bake 20-25 minutes or until the eggs are set. Serve. To store, keep refrigerated for up to 5 days.

Prep Time: 20 Minutes

Cook Time: 30 Minutes

Servings: 2

Ingredients

- 2/3 cup cream cheese, room temperature (160 g/ 5.6 oz)
- 2 tbsp pumpkin puree (30 g/ 1.1 oz) - you can make your own
- 1 large egg yolk
- 2 tbsp Erythritol or Swerve (20 g/ 0.7 oz)
- 1/2 tsp pumpkin pie spice - you can make your own

Dough:

- 3/4 cup shredded mozzarella (85 g/ 3 oz) - use low-moisture, part-skim, shredded mozzarella cheese; not fresh mozzarella.
- 1/3 cup almond flour (33 g/ 1.2 oz)

Instructions

1. Preheat the oven to 200 °C/ 400 °F (fan). Prepare the filling. Place the softened cream cheese, pumpkin puree, egg yolk, Erythritol and pumpkin pie spice in a bowl.Keto Pumpkin Cheesecake Breakfast Pockets

2. Mix until well combined. Set aside.Keto Pumpkin Cheesecake Breakfast Pockets

3. Place the shredded mozzarella in another bowl and microwave for 30-60 seconds, or melt on the stove over a low heat.Keto Pumpkin Cheesecake Breakfast Pockets

4. Mix in the almond flour.Keto Pumpkin Cheesecake Breakfast Pockets

5. Using a fork, combine well until you create dough.Keto Pumpkin Cheesecake Breakfast Pockets

6. Roll the dough out between 2 sheets of parchment paper until very thin (I used a silicon mat and silicon rolling pin).Keto Pumpkin Cheesecake Breakfast Pockets

7. Scoop the pumpkin cheesecake filling in the centre of the dough.Keto Pumpkin Cheesecake Breakfast Pockets

8. Fold over like an envelope and seal the dough. Pumpkin Cheesecake Breakfast Pockets

9. Poke some holes for releasing the steam while baking. Transfer onto a baking sheet lined with parchment paper.Keto Pumpkin Cheesecake Breakfast Pockets

10. Bake for about 15 minutes or until golden brown on top.Keto Pumpkin Cheesecake Breakfast Pockets

11. When done, remove from the oven and let it cool down for a few minutes. Slice and serve!Keto Pumpkin Cheesecake Breakfast Pockets

12. Optionally, dust with some powdered Erythritol or Swerve, and cinnamon. The pockets can be stored in the fridge for up to 3 days. Reheat before serving or eat cold.

Prep Time: 20 Minutes

Cook Time: 25 Minutes

Servings: 2

Ingredients

- 170 g gluten-free sausage meat (6 oz)
- 2 tbsp extra virgin olive oil or ghee (30 ml)
- 2 cups diced turnips (260 g/ 9.2 oz)
- 1/2 small yellow onion, chopped (35 g/ 1.2 oz)
- 2 cloves garlic, minced
- 1/4 tsp sea salt, or to taste
- 1/8 tsp black pepper, or to taste
- 1/2 cup drained kimchi (70 g/ 2.5 oz)
- 2 tbsp minced chives, for garnish

Instructions

1. In a large pan over medium-high heat, brown the sausage crumbling with the back of a wooden spoon for about 5 minutes.

2. Once browned remove the sausage and add the olive oil to the skillet.

3. Low-Carb Kimchi Sausage Breakfast Hash

4. Once the oil is hot, add the turnips, cooking for about 5 minutes before adding in the onion and garlic. Cook for an additional 5-7 minutes until the turnips are golden and tender.

5. Low-Carb Kimchi Sausage Breakfast Hash

6. Add the sausage back to the skillet and season with salt and pepper to taste. Serve with kimchi and chives. Store leftovers in an airtight container in the refrigerator for up to 4 days.

Prep Time: 20 Minutes

Cook Time: 25 Minutes

Servings: 2

Ingredients

- 2 tbsp ghee (30 g/ 1.1 oz) - I used my Golden Ghee
- 250 g asparagus (8.8 oz)
- 1 pack spinach (200 g/ 7.1 oz)
- sea salt and black pepper, to taste
- 4 gluten-free sausages (240 g/ 8.5 oz)
- 4 large eggs
- 1 cup Pink Sauerkraut or White Sauerkraut (142 g/ 5 oz)
- 1/2 large avocado, sliced (100 g/ 3.5 oz)
- 1 tbsp extra virgin olive oil (15 ml)
- 1 tbsp chopped parsley

Instructions

1. Chop the asparagus, or keep whole spears if you like(. I used green and purple asparagus ends that I had left

after making fermented asparagus.)Keto Superfood All Day Breakfast Skillet

2. Place the asparagus in a hot skillet greased with half of the ghee. Season with a pinch of salt and pepper. Cook over a medium heat for about 5 minutes.

3. Add the fresh spinach and cook for another 30-60 seconds or until wilted. Superfood All Day Breakfast Skillet

4. Take off the heat. Transfer the content of the skillet to a plate.Superfood All Day Breakfast Skillet

5. Grease the same skillet with the remaining ghee. Add the sausages and cook until browned on all sides and cooked through. Remove from the skillet and set aside.

6. Finally, fry the eggs over a medium-high heat, until the egg whites are set and opaque and the egg yolks are still runny. Take off the heat. Superfood All Day Breakfast Skillet

7. Move the fried eggs on the side. Add the cooked asparagus, spinach and sausages. Add the sauerkraut and top with sliced avocado.

8. Drizzle with olive oil. Garnish with fresh parsley and season with salt and pepper to taste. Eat immediately or refrigerate for up to a day.

Prep Time: 15 Minutes

Cook Time: 15 Minutes

Servings: 2

Ingredients

- 3 large eggs, separated
- 1/4 tsp cream of tartar or apple cider vinegar
- 2 tbsp powdered Erythritol or Swerve (20 g/ 0.7 oz) or 5-10 drops Stevia
- 1/2 tsp fresh lemon zest
- 2 tbsp coconut flour (16 g/ 0.5 oz)
- 1 tsp ghee or coconut oil

Optional:

- serve with full-fat yogurt, sour cream or creamed coconut milk
- 1/4 cup berry sauce (recipe below)

Berry sauce:

- 1/2 cup blackberries, fresh or frozen (75 g/ 2.6 oz)
- 1/2 cup wild blueberries, fresh or frozen (75 g/ 2.6 oz)

- 3 tbsp water

- 2 tbsp powdered Erythritol or Swerve (20 g/ 0.7 oz) or 5-10 drops Stevia

- 1/4 tsp vanilla powder or 1 tsp sugar-free vanilla extract

- 1 tbsp fresh lemon juice

- 2 tsp ground chia seeds or 1 tbsp whole chia seeds

Instructions

1. Start by preparing the berry sauce. Place the blackberries and blueberries in a saucepan. Add water, Erythritol, vanilla powder and lemon juice. Cook over a medium heat until the berries start to soften. Take off the heat and mix in the ground or whole chia seeds.Keto Lemon Soufflé & Berry Pancake

2. Let it sit for 10-15 minutes to thicken. Meanwhile, prepare the pancake. Set the oven to broil at 200 °C/ 400 °F (fan assisted), or 220 °C/ 425 °F (conventional). Separate the egg whites from the egg yolks. Using a fork, mix the egg yolks.Keto Lemon Soufflé & Berry Pancake

3. Start beating the egg whites on medium-low speed. Continue for about 2 minutes until the whites become foamy. Then, add the cream of tartar (or apple cider vinegar). Add powdered Erythritol, a tablespoon at a time. Keep beating until the egg whites create soft peaks. Lemon Soufflé & Berry Pancake

4. Add the lemon zest and egg yolks and gently fold into the egg whites using a silicon spatula.

5. Keto Lemon Soufflé & Berry Pancake

6. Sift in the coconut flour and slowly combine with the egg mixture without deflating the egg whites.Keto Lemon Soufflé & Berry Pancake

7. Spread the pancake batter in a hot skillet greased with ghee (I used an 8-inch skillet). Cook on low heat for about 5 minutes until the bottom of the pancake starts to brown. Remove from the burner and place in the oven under the broiler for 3-5 minutes or until lightly browned.Keto Lemon Soufflé & Berry Pancake

8. Serve with the berry sauce on top (about 1/4 cup/ 60 ml per pancake). Reserve the remaining berry sauce for more pancakes and store in an airtight container for up to a week.

9. Tip: Instead of the berry sauce, you can try Sugar-free Amarenata (just skip the lemon zest in the pancake

and use vanilla extract instead) or sauce made with
any other berries.

Prep Time: 10 Minutes

Cook Time: 30 Minutes

Servings: 2

Ingredients

Cheese filling:

- 2/3 cup cream cheese (160 g/ 5.6 oz)
- 1 large egg yolk
- 2 tbsp powdered Erythritol, Swerve or Allulose (20 g/ 0.7 oz)
- 1/2 tsp fine fresh lemon zest
- 1/2 tsp sugar-free vanilla extract

Danish pancake:

- 3 large egg whites
- 2 large egg yolks
- 1/2 tsp lemon juice or 1/4 tsp cream of tartar
- 2 tbsp powdered Erythritol, Swerve or Allulose (20 g/ 0.7 oz)
- 2 tbsp coconut flour (16 g/ 0.6 oz)

- 1/3 cup almond flour (33 g/ 1.2 oz) or 1 1/2 tbsp coconut flour (12 g/ 0.4 oz)
- 1 tbsp ghee or virgin coconut oil (15 ml)
- 1/4 cup frozen or fresh wild blueberries (38 g/ 1.3 oz)

Optional:

- powdered Erythritol, Swerve or Allulose for dusting

Instructions

1. Preheat the oven to 150 °C/ 300 °F (fan assisted), or 170 °C/ 340 °F (conventional). Separate the egg whites from the egg yolks.Low-Carb Blueberry Skillet Danish
2. To make the filling: Combine the cream cheese with 1 egg yolk, fresh lemon zest, vanilla, and 2 tbsp sweetener (Erythritol, Swerve or Allulose).Low-Carb Blueberry Skillet Danish
3. To make the pancake: To the bowl with the egg whites add the lemon juice (or use 1/4 tsp cream of tartar). Using an electric mixer or a hand whisk, start whisking the egg whites and add in the remaining 2 tablespoons of sweetener. Keep beating until stiff peaks form.Low-Carb Blueberry Skillet Danish

4. Fold the remaining 2 egg yolks into the mixture using a silicone spatula.Low-Carb Blueberry Skillet Danish

5. Sift in the almond flour and coconut flour and gently combine with the egg white mixture without deflating it (check recipe tips for nut-free options).Low-Carb Blueberry Skillet Danish

6. Grease an ovenproof 8-inch (20-cm) skillet with ghee (or coconut oil) and heat it over medium heat. Pour in the fluffy pancake mixture, and then cook on low heat for 1 minute. Spoon the filling in the middle of the pancake and spread evenly, leaving about an inch (2.5 cm) on the sides.Low-Carb Blueberry Skillet Danish

7. Add the blueberries (fresh or frozen), transfer the skillet to the oven, and bake for 20 to 25 minutes, until the pancake is golden and the filling is set.Low-Carb Blueberry Skillet Danish

8. Optionally, dust with powdered sweetener. Eat warm or cold. This recipe makes two regular breakfast servings or up to four dessert servings. Store in the fridge for up to 3 days.

Prep Time: 10 Minutes

Cook Time: 20 Minutes

Servings: 2

Ingredients

- 2 tbsp extra virgin avocado oil or ghee (30 ml)
- 1/2 medium yellow onion, chopped (50 g/ 1.8 oz)
- 2 cloves garlic, diced
- 2 tbsp tomato paste (30 g/ 1.1 oz)
- 2 cans tuna, drained (255 g/ 9 oz)
- 1 tsp turmeric
- 1/2 tsp ground cumin
- 1/2 tsp paprika
- 1/2 cup filtered water or brine from tuna (120 ml/ 4 fl oz)
- sea salt and ground pepper, to taste
- 2-4 tbsp chopped cilantro
- 6 large eggs
- 2 tbsp extra virgin olive oil to drizzle (30 ml)

Optional:

- 1/4 cup shredded cheddar cheese or goat's cheese

Optional:

- lime wedges to serve

Instructions

1. Prepare all the ingredients. Grease a large skillet with 2 tablespoons of avocado and sauté onions for about 5 minutes. Add the garlic and cook for 1 more minute.Low-Carb Tuna Shakshuka

2. When the onions become fragrant and lightly golden, add the tomatoes paste. After 1 minute, add tuna and stir well. Add all the spices, salt and pepper, water, and then stir.

3. Bring to a boil, then reduce the heat and let it simmer for about 10 minutes, or until the sauce has thickened. Add cilantro chopped and stir. You can reserve some cilantro for garnish.Low-Carb Tuna Shakshuka

4. Using a spoon or a ladle, make 6 wells in the skillet and carefully crack the eggs inside each. Once the egg whites seem to be mostly cooked through (about 8 minutes) cover the skillet to cook the top of the eggs,

checking periodically to ensure the yolks don't get overcooked.

5. Optionally, sprinkle with cheddar cheese and let it cook for another 3-4 minutes.Low-Carb Tuna Shakshuka

6. Remove from the heat and garnish with salt and fresh cilantro. Eat while still warm.

11. Creamy Mushroom Chicken Skillet

Prep Time: 15 Minutes

Cook Time: 30 Minutes

Servings:

Ingredients

- 2 medium skinless chicken breasts (400 g/ 14.1 oz)
- sea salt and pepper, to taste
- 3 tbsp ghee or avocado oil (45 ml)
- 1 small yellow onion, diced (70 g/ 2.5 oz)
- 2 cloves garlic, minced
- 2 cups sliced brown mushrooms (144 g/ 5 oz)
- 1/2 cup creme fraiche or sour cream (120 g/ 4.2 oz)
- 3/4 cups chicken stock or bone broth (180 ml/ 6 fl oz)
- 1 tbsp fresh chopped herbs such as parsley, thyme, basil, and/or chives)
- Optional: serve with zucchini noodles - here's how to prepare them

Instructions

1. Season the chicken breasts with salt and pepper from both sides. If the breasts are too thick, flatten the thickest parts with a mallet.

2. Grease a skillet with 1 tbsp of ghee or avocado oil. Add the chicken breasts and cook on medium-high for about 5 minutes without moving, or until golden brown.

3. Flip on the other side, cook for about a minute, and then reduce the heat to medium. Cover with a lid and cook for about 10 minutes, or until the thickest part of the chicken is cooked through. (If you use a meat thermometer, the temperature should reach about 75 °C/ 165 °F.) Remove from the skillet and set aside.Keto Creamy Mushroom Chicken Skillet

4. Grease the skillet where you cooked the chicken with the remaining ghee. Dice the onion and mince the garlic. Add the onion to the skillet and cook on medium-high until fragrant, for about 5 minutes.

5. Meanwhile, slice the mushrooms. Add the sliced mushrooms and cook for 2 to 3 minutes mixing a few times. Creamy Mushroom Chicken Skillet

6. Add the stock and bring to a boil. Cook for a few minutes, until the mushrooms are tender. If you're

using zucchini noodles as a side, this is when I add the chopped zucchini cores to the skillet. If you want your sauce to be thick and creamy, cook for a little longer to reduce it.Keto Creamy Mushroom Chicken Skillet

7. Add the creme fraiche (or sour cream) and stir to combine. Cook for another 2 minutes. Add the fresh chopped herbs.

8. Finally, add back the chicken breasts and cook for a few minutes just to heat through. Creamy Mushroom Chicken Skillet

9. Optionally, serve with zucchini noodles — here's how to prepare them, or with shirataki noodles for a lower carb option (here's how to prepare shirataki noodles).

Prep Time: 10 Minutes

Cook Time: 25 Minutes

Servings: 1

Ingredients

Caesar salad dressing:

- 1 cup paleo mayonnaise (240 ml/ 8 fl oz) - you can make your own
- 3 cloves garlic, crushed
- 3 jarred anchovy fillets, finely chopped or 1 tbsp anchovy paste
- 2 tbsp fresh lemon juice (30 ml)
- 1 tbsp Dijon mustard
- 1 tbsp Worcestershire sauce or coconut aminos (15 ml)
- 4 tbsp grated Parmesan cheese or any Italian-style hard cheese (20 g/ 0.7 oz)

Caesar salad:

- 1 skinless chicken breast (170 g/ 6 oz)

- 1/2 head of Romaine lettuce or any lettuce of choice (150 g/ 5.3 oz)
- 2 tbsp grated or flaked Parmesan cheese (10 g/ 0.4 oz)
- 2 tbsp prepared Caesar Salad Dressing (30 ml)
- 5 to 7 pork rinds, crushed into smaller pieces (10 g/ 0.4 oz)

Instructions

1. First, prepare the Caesar Salad Dressing. Peel and crush the garlic. If using whole anchovies, chop them as finely as you can to create paste. Place all of the ingredients in a mason jar. Cover with a lid and shake until well combined. Shake until well combined. For smoother texture you can place the ingredients in a food processor and process until smooth.

2. Note: The recipe will make enough dressing for 10 servings. Per each serving you'll only need 2 tablespoons (30 ml). Store the remaining salad dressing in the jar sealed in the fridge for up to a week.Caesar Salad with Zero-Carb Croutons

3. To cook the chicken breast, rub the chicken with one teaspoon of olive oil or ghee and season with salt and pepper. Heat another teaspoon of oil in a skillet over a

medium heat. Place chicken breasts in and cook until edges are opaque, for about 10 minutes.

4. Flip the chicken breast and then cover the pan, lower the heat and cook for another 10 minutes. Once cooked, take off the heat and let it rest for 5 minutes before slicing.Caesar Salad with Zero-Carb Croutons

5. To assemble, tear the lettuce into smaller pieces and place in a salad bowl. Top with sliced chicken, parmesan cheese and 2 tablespoons (30 ml) of the prepared salad dressing. Top with pork rinds broken into smaller pieces. (Or instead of pork rinds you can use Chicken Cracklings.)Caesar Salad with Zero-Carb Croutons

6. Eat immediately.Caesar Salad with Zero-Carb Croutons

7. To store, refrigerate for up to a day (without the croutons as they should always be added just before serving).

Prep Time: 15 Minutes

Cook Time: 45 Minutes

Servings: 4

Ingredients

Chicken:

- 1.5 lbs chicken breast, cut into 1-inch (2 cm) cubes (680 g)
- 3 tbsp olive oil (45 ml)
- 2 tbsp lemon juice (30 ml)
- 1 tbsp red wine vinegar
- 1 tbsp dried oregano
- 1 tsp onion powder
- 1 tsp garlic powder
- 1/2 tsp salt
- 1/4 tsp pepper

Greek Salsa:

- 1 cucumber, diced (200 g/ 7.1 oz)
- 1 cup cherry tomatoes, sliced in half (130 g/ 5 oz)
- 1/2 cup diced red onion (80 g/ 2.8 oz)

- 1/3 cup kalamata olive slices (60 g/ 2.1 oz)
- 3 tbsp olive oil (45 ml)
- 1 tbsp red wine vinegar
- 1 tsp dried oregano
- 4 oz feta cheese (113 g)
- Salt, to taste

Tzatziki:

- 8 oz full-fat Greek yogurt (227 g)
- 1/2 cucumber, minced (100 g/ 3.5 oz)
- 2 cloves garlic, minced
- zest of 1 lemon
- 1 tbsp lemon juice
- 2 tbsp minced fresh dill
- salt and pepper, to taste

Optionally serve with:

- 3 cups cauliflower rice (360 g/ 12.7 oz) + 2.7 g net carbs per serving

Instructions

1. Cut the chicken into 1-inch (2 cm) cubes. Place in a sealable container with the remaining marinade

ingredients. Toss to coat. Let the chicken marinate for at least 30 minutes. Greek Chicken Bowls

2. While the chicken is marinating make the salsa by dicing the cucumber, halving the tomatoes, and dicing the onion. Place into a medium bowl with the olives and toss with olive oil, vinegar, and oregano. Gently stir in the feta cheese. Taste for salt and add more if needed. Greek Chicken Bowls

3. For the Tzatziki combine the yogurt with the minced cucumber, minced garlic, lemon zest and juice, and dill in a medium bowl. Season with salt and pepper to your taste.

4. Once the chicken has marinated heat a large skillet over medium high heat. Add the chicken along with the marinade in a single layer. Cook 4 minutes per side or until each side is golden and the chicken is cooked through. Remove from pan and set aside. Greek Chicken Bowls

5. Optional if using cauli-rice: Add the cauliflower rice (here's how to make cauli-rice) to the same skillet scraping up any stuck on pieces of marinade from the bottom. Cook just until soft.

6. To assemble divide the chicken and cauliflower rice between four containers. Layer in the salsa and top

with Tzatziki. These bowls will keep for 4-5 days in the refrigerator.

Prep Time: 15 Minutes

Cook Time: 30 Minutes

Servings: 1

Ingredients

- 2 skinless chicken breasts (500 g/ 1.1 lb)
- 2 tbsp taco seasoning (15 g/ 0.5 oz)
- 3 tbsp extra virgin avocado oil or ghee (30 ml)
- 1 each medium red, yellow and green peppers (120 g/ 4.2 oz each, 360 g/ 12.7 oz total)
- 1/2 small red onion (30 g/ 1.1 oz)
- 1 large avocado (200 g/ 7.1 oz)
- 4 cups baby spinach leaves (120 g/ 4.2 oz)
- 1 cup sour cream (240 ml/ 8 fl oz)
- 4 sprigs fresh cilantro
- 4 tbsp extra virgin olive oil to drizzle (60 ml)

Instructions

1. Prepare all the ingredients. Mix the taco seasoning spices if you are making your own.Low-Carb Chicken Fajita Lunch Bowl

2. Lay the chicken breasts out on a sheet of baking paper, drizzle them with 1 tbsp avocado oil and then sprinkle them with 1 tablespoon of seasoned rub per each side.

3. Massage the rub into the chicken and then cook it over high heat on a BBQ or grill plate until seared and caramelised on the outside, lower the heat and finish cooking until the juices run clear.

4. Remove and cover loosely with foil to rest while you finish preparing the roasted vegetables.

Low-Carb Chicken Fajita Lunch Bowl

5. Peel and cut the onion into wedges, separate the layers. Core and seed the peppers and cut into chunky strips.

6. Heat 2 tablespoons of avocado oil in a large frying pan and cook the peppers and red onions until softened and slightly charred.

7. Chicken Fajita Lunch Bowl

8. Slice the chicken across the grain into strips.

9. Chicken Fajita Lunch Bowl

10. Layer the bowls with spinach, roasted vegetables and sliced chicken and then top with avocado and sour cream. Garnish with coriander and drizzle with olive oil, 1 tablespoon per bowl.

11. You can store the chicken and the cooked peppers in a covered container in the fridge for up to 4 days. Don't store the avocado, as it will brown. Cut the avocado fresh before you eat it.

Prep Time: 20 Minutes

Cook Time: 20 Minutes

Servings: 1

Ingredients

Lunch bowl:

- 2 boneless mackerel fillets (225 g/ 8 oz)
- 1 1/2 cups broccoli (137 g/ 4.8 oz)
- 1/2 small yellow onion (35 g/ 1.2 oz)
- 1 tbsp ghee, butter or coconut oil (15 g/ 0.5 oz)
- 1/3 cup diced red bell pepper (50 g/ 1.8 oz)
- 2 pieces sun-dried tomatoes, chopped (6 g/ 0.2 oz)
- small handful of almonds (20 g/ 0.7 oz)
- 4 tbsp mashed avocado or keto hummus (58 g/ 2 oz)

Marinade:

- 1 tbsp grated ginger (6 g/ 0.2 oz)
- 1 tbsp fresh lime or lemon juice (15 ml)
- 3 tbsp extra virgin olive oil (45 ml)
- 1 tbsp coconut aminos (15 ml)
- 1/4 tsp sea salt, or to taste

- 1/8 tsp cracked black pepper

Instructions

1. Preheat the oven to 200 °C/ 400 °F (fan assisted). Line a baking tray with greaseproof paper. Rub half the dressing on the mackerel fillets (non skin side).
2. Crispy Ginger Mackerel Lunch Bowl
3. Place the mackerel fillets on the baking tray skin side up and roast for 10 - 12 minutes until crispy, or to your liking. (If you're short on time, skip the marinating and simply bake in the oven.)
4. Place the almonds on a separate baking tray and roast in the oven for 6 minutes until golden. Remove from the oven and allow to cool before chopping them.
5. Crispy Ginger Mackerel Keto Lunch Bowl
6. Steam the broccoli florets in a pan of water for about 5 minutes, until al dente. Roughly chop the broccoli or gently crush with a fork.
7. Crispy Ginger Mackerel Lunch Bowl
8. Heat 1 tbsp of ghee, butter or coconut oil in a pan. Add the onion and peppers. Fry for 2-3 minutes on a medium heat until soft.

9. Stir through the broccoli and sun dried tomatoes until warm. Turn off the heat.

10. Crispy Ginger Mackerel Keto Lunch Bowl

11. Mix through the remaining dressing and top with chopped roasted almonds and avocado cream or keto hummus. Tastes best when served fresh but can be stored in the fridge for 3 days.

Prep Time: 15 Minutes

Cook Time: 20 Minutes

Servings: 1

Ingredients

- 1 tuna steak (120 g/ 4.2 oz) - or use tinned, drained tuna
- 1 tsp sesame seeds
- pinch of sea salt
- 1 tsp ghee, butter or virgin coconut oil
- 1/2 avocado, sliced (100 g/ 3.5 oz)
- 10 pitted black olives (30 g/ 1.1 oz)
- 1 tbsp mayonnaise (15 g/ 0.5 oz) - you can make your own mayo
- 1/2 medium cucumber, sliced (70 g/ 2.5 oz)
- 6 quails eggs or 1 large egg
- 1/4 small red onion, finely sliced (15 g/ 0.5 oz)
- 10 walnut halves (20 g/ 0.7 oz)
- 1 tbsp extra virgin olive oil (15 ml)
- large handful of watercress (50 g/ 1.8 oz)

Instructions

1. Preheat the oven to 180 °C/ 355 °F (fan assisted) 200 °C/ 400 °F (conventional). Wash and dry the watercress.

2. Place the walnuts on a baking tray and roast in the oven for 6-8 minutes until golden. Remove from the oven and allow to cool.

3. Speedy Low-Carb Tuna Lunch Bowl

4. Coat the tuna with sesame seeds, ghee and a pinch of salt. If using tinned tuna, simply sprinkle the sesame seeds over the salad in the end.

5. Heat a griddle pan and fry the tuna to your liking - 1 1/2 minutes per side for pink, up to 3 minutes per side for well done. Remove from the heat and allow to cool slightly before slicing.

6. Speedy Low-Carb Tuna Lunch Bowl

7. Boil the quail eggs for 2-3 minutes (or about 10 minutes for large eggs). Plunge into cold water before peeling.

8. Speedy Low-Carb Tuna Lunch Bowl

9. Slice the rest of ingredients.

10. Speedy Low-Carb Tuna Lunch Bowl

11. Place the watercress in bowl and add olives, halved quail eggs, avocado, walnuts and drizzle with 1 tbsp of

olive oil and top with 1 tbsp of mayonnaise. Optionally, garnish with ground black pepper.

12. Speedy Low-Carb Tuna Lunch Bowl
13. Tastes the best when served fresh, but can be stored in the fridge for 1 day.

Prep Time: 5 Minutes

Cook Time: 5 Minutes

Servings: 1

Ingredients

- 2 medium avocados or 1 extra large avocado, seed removed (300 g/ 10.6 oz)
- 1 1/2 cup cooked chicken (210 g/ 7.4 oz)
- 1/4 cup paleo mayonnaise or creme fraiche (58 g/ 2 oz) - you can make your own
- 2 tbsp sour cream or cream cheese or more mayo for dairy-free (24 g/ 0.8 oz)
- 1 tsp thyme, dried
- 1 tsp paprika
- 1/2 tsp onion powder
- 1/2 tsp garlic powder
- 1/4 tsp cayenne pepper
- 2 tbsp fresh lemon juice
- 1/4 tsp salt or more to taste

Instructions

1. Cut or shred the cooked chicken into small pieces.Cajun Chicken Stuffed Avocado

2. Add the mayo, sour cream, thyme, paprika, onion powder, garlic powder and cayenne pepper.Cajun Chicken Stuffed Avocado

3. Add lemon juice and season with salt to taste.Cajun Chicken Stuffed Avocado

4. Combine well. Scoop the middle of the avocado out leaving 1/2 to 1 inch of the avocado flesh. Cut the scooped avocado into small pieces.

5. Place the chopped avocado into the bowl with the chicken and mix until well combined. Fill each avocado half with the chicken & avocado mixture.

6. Eat immediately or store in the fridge for up to a day. The chicken filling can be stored in the fridge in a sealed jar for up to 3 days.

Prep Time: 5 Minutes

Cook Time: 40 Minutes

Servings: 6

Ingredients

- 1 large celeriac, peeled (250 g/ 8.8 oz)
- 1 small cauliflower (400 g/ 14.1 oz)
- 4 garlic cloves
- 4 tbsp extra virgin olive oil or melted butter (60 ml/ 2 fl oz)
- 2 tsp dried oregano
- 3 tbsp fresh rosemary or 1 tsp dried rosemary
- 1 tsp fresh thyme or 1/2 tsp died thyme
- 1 cup crumbled feta cheese (150 g/ 5.3 oz)
- 1/2 tsp sea salt
- 1/4 tsp cracked black pepper
- fresh oregano or herbs of choice for garnish

Instructions

1. Preheat the oven to 190 °C/ 375 °F (fan assisted) 210 °C/ 410 °F. Cop the celeriac into about about 2 cm/ 0.8 inch cubes. Cut the celeriac into small florets. Peel and finely chop the garlic.

2. Add the chopped celeriac, cauliflower and garlic cloves to a baking tray. Add the herbs and butter or olive oil, season with salt and pepper and toss well.

3. Roast "Notatoes" with Garlic and Feta

4. Roast in the oven for 30 - 35 minutes until golden. Top with fresh oregano and feta.

5. Roast "Notatoes" with Garlic and Feta

6. Tastes best when served fresh, but can be stored in the fridge for up to 3 days.

7. Roast "Notatoes" with Garlic and Feta

8. Enjoy as a side dish or a light dinner, or double the serving for a full satisfying meal.

Prep Time: 15 Minutes

Cook Time: 25 Minutes

Servings: 2

Ingredients

- 4 slices raw bacon (120 g/ 4.2 oz) - or 64 g/ 2.2 oz crisped up
- 10-14 asparagus spears, woody ends removed (100 g/ 3.5 oz)
- 1 tbsp butter or ghee (14 g/ 0.5 oz)
- 2 large eggs
- 1 small head lettuce such as little gem (100 g/ 3.5 oz)
- 1/2 large avocado, sliced (100 g/ 3.5 oz)
- 1/3 cup crumpled feta cheese (50 g/ 1.8 oz)
- 1/3 cup cherry tomatoes, halved (50 g/ 1.8 oz)
- 2 tsp chopped chives or spring onion
- 1/4 cup flaked almonds, preferably toasted (23 g/ 0.8 oz)

Dressing:

- 3 tbsp extra virgin olive oil (45 ml/ 1.5 fl oz)

- 1 tsp Dijon mustard

- 2 tsp red wine vinegar

- sea salt and black pepper, to taste

Instructions

1. Crisp up the bacon in the oven or in a skillet. Oven is better for large batches. If you're only cooking 4 slices it's faster to cook in a lightly greased skillet.

2. Skillet: In a frying pan, fry the bacon rashers for 2 minutes per side until crisp. I dry fried them but you can add a touch of olive oil or ghee if you prefer to prevent sticking. All depends on your pan. Drain on a sheet of kitchen paper.

3. Oven: Preheat the oven to 190 °C/ 375 °F. Line a baking tray with baking paper. Lay the bacon strips out flat on the baking paper, leaving space so they don't overlap. Place the tray in the oven and cook for about 10-15 minutes until golden brown. The time depends on the thickness of the bacon slices. When done, remove from the oven and set aside to cool down. Store any leftover bacon in the fridge for up to 4 days.

4. Slice the tomatoes and avocado. Chop the lettuce.Bacon, Egg & Asparagus Keto Bowl

5. Prepare the dressing my mixing the olive oil, mustard, vinegar, salt and pepper together in a small bowl.

6. Bacon, Egg & Asparagus Keto Bowl

7. Place water in the bottom of a steamer pan. Steam the asparagus for 5 – 8 minutes depending on the thickness of the asparagus until el dente. Remove from the pan, coat in 1 tablespoon of butter and chop into chunks.

8. Bacon, Egg & Asparagus Keto Bowl

9. While the asparagus is cooking, boil the eggs to your liking. 3 minutes for soft boiled up to 10 minutes for hard boiled. Run under cold water before peeling off the shell.

10. Toss the lettuce through the tomatoes, crispy bacon and dressing. Top with boiled egg, feta, avocado, asparagus, chives, and almonds.

11. Bacon, Egg & Asparagus Keto Bowl

12. Best eaten fresh but can be stored in the fridge for a day.

Prep Time: 15 Minutes

Cook Time: 25 Minutes

Servings: 6

Ingredients

Raspberry Curd:

- 2 cups frozen raspberries (300 g/ 10.5 oz)
- 1 tbsp lemon juice (15 ml)
- 1 tsp fresh lemon zest
- 1/2 cup powdered Erythritol or Swerve (80 g/ 2.8 oz)
- 15-20 drops liquid stevia
- 4 large egg yolks
- 1 tsp gelatine powder, bloomed in 2 tbsp of cold water
- 1 tbsp butter, ghee or virgin coconut oil (14 g/ 0.5 oz)
- Meringue
- 4 large egg whites
- 1/3 cup powdered Erythritol or Swerve (53 g/ 1.9 oz)
- 1/4 tsp cream of tartar

Garnish:

- 4-6 freeze-dried raspberries

Instructions

1. Place the raspberries, stevia and lemon zest into a saucepan.
2. Add lemon juice and bring to the boil. Simmer for five minutes.
3. Place the raspberry mixture in a fine mesh sieve and push through until smooth, discarding the seeds.
4. Return the raspberry puree to your cleaned saucepan, add the sweetener and set aside.
5. Separate the egg yolks and whites. Whisk the egg yolks and then add the bloomed gelatine. Whisk well until no lumps remain.
6. Add the egg yolk mixture to the raspberries and mix well.
7. Heat over a medium heat until he mixture starts to bubble, stirring continuously. Once you see bubbles, remove from the heart, add butter and stir until melted.
8. Set your glasses, jars or ramekins out (I used 4 oz/ 120 ml jars). Pour the raspberry curd evenly into your jars and place in refrigerator to set for approx. 1.5 hours. Preheat oven to 175 °C/ 350 °F (fan assisted), or 195 °C/ 380 °F (conventional).

9. Place egg whites in the bowl of your electric mixer and beat with a whisk attachment. Slowly add cream of tartar to whisking egg whites. One teaspoon at a time, add the sweetener, making sure to beat well in-between additions. Whisk until stiff peaks form. Raspberry Meringue Pots

10. Remove set curd from fridge and spoon meringue on top, adding height and swirls to taste.

11. Place on a baking tray and cook for 15 - 18 minutes, until the meringue is browned to your taste.

12. Remove and let cool. Crumble the freeze-dried raspberries on top for garnish.

13. Return to fridge until ready to eat. Eat immediately if not able to cover. Otherwise, store covered in the refrigerator, for up to two days.

Prep Time: 30 Minutes

Cook Time: 45 Minutes

Servings: 3

Ingredients

Fish cakes:

- 2 cups cauliflower rice (240 g/ 8.5 oz) - here's how to "rice" cauliflower
- 4 tbsp ghee or virgin coconut oil (60 g/ 2.1 oz)
- 1 clove garlic, minced
- 800 g white fish fillets, skinless and boneless, such as cod or haddock (1.76 lb)
- 1 tsp sea salt, or to taste
- 1/2 tsp freshly ground black pepper
- 1 tsp fresh lemon zest
- 1 tsp ground cumin
- 2 tbsp freshly chopped parsley
- 1 large spring onion, chopped (28 g/ 1 oz)
- 2 large eggs

- 1/2 cup almond flour or grated Parmesan cheese (50 g/ 1.8 oz)
- 4 tbsp flax meal (28 g/ 1 oz)

Aioli:

- 1/2 cup Homemade Mayonnaise (110 g/ 3.9 oz)
- 2 cloves garlic, minced

Instructions

1. Start by cooking the cauliflower rice (here's how to make cauliflower rice). Grease a small saucepan with 1 tablespoon of ghee and add 1 clove of minced garlic. Cook over a medium heat for just about 30 seconds or until fragrant, add the cauli-rice and season with a pinch of salt. Stir and cook for 5-7 minutes, until crisp-tender. When done, take off the heat and set aside. Fish Cakes with Aioli

2. Cook the fish. Use a paper towel to pat dry the fillets from all sides and season with some salt and pepper. Heat a large pan greased with a tablespoon of ghee over a medium-high heat. Once hot, add the fish and cook for 2-3 minutes without flipping it (time depends on the thickness of the fillet).

3. When ready to flip, use a spatula and cook it for another 2-3 minutes. When cooked, the fillets should be opaque and flaky. Do not overcook the fish or it will get too dry. Use a spatula to transfer the fish into a bowl and set aside to cool down for 5-10 minutes. Fish Cakes with Aioli

4. Add the cooked cauliflower rice, freshly grated lemon zest, ground cumin, chopped parsley, spring onion, eggs, almond flour and flax meal. Season with the remaining salt and pepper and mix until well combined. Fish Cakes with Aioli

5. To make the patties, use a 1/4 measuring cup. Spoon the mixture into the cup and use a spoon to press it in until flat. Turn it over and empty onto a chopping board. Use your hands if you need to reshape the patties. Repeat with the remaining mixture until you get 18 patties. Fish Cakes with Aioli

6. Heat a large frypan greased with a tablespoon of ghee over a medium-high heat. Once hot, reduce the heat to medium and place the patties in the frypan. Cook for 3-5 minutes on each side, until golden. Do not try to flip the patties before they are ready or you will break the crust (you can test that by moving them slightly with a spatula). Work in batches - do not

overfill the pan and grease as needed.Keto Fish Cakes with Aioli

7. Prepare the aioli by mixing the mayonnaise and minced garlic. Fish Cakes with AioliServe the patties with aioli and low-carb sides or salads such as my Paleo Spinach Tabbouleh, Low-Carb CousCous or Quick & Easy Guacamole. To store, let them cool down and refrigerate for up to 3 days - or freeze for up to 3 months.

Prep Time: 10 Minutes

Cook Time: 30 Minutes

Servings: 4

Ingredients

Turkey patties:

- 500 g turkey, ground (1.1 lb)
- 1/2 cup almond flour (50 g/ 1.8 oz)
- 1 large egg 2 cloves garlic, crushed
- 1 small hot chili pepper, chopped
- 2 tsp Dijon mustard
- 2 tbsp lemon juice (30 ml)
- 2 tbsp chopped parsley
- 2 tbsp chopped basil
- 1/2 tsp sea salt
- ground black pepper, to taste
- 2 medium spring onions, finely sliced (30 g/ 1.1 oz)
- 2 tbsp ghee or lard (30 ml)
- Cucumber salsa:
- 2 medium cucumbers (500 g/17.6 oz)

- 1 jalapeño pepper, halved and deseeded (15 g/ 0.5 oz)
- 1 clove garlic, crushed
- 1 tablespoon apple cider vinegar (15 ml)
- 1 tablespoon chopped fresh dill
- 2 tablespoons extra virgin olive oil (30 ml)
- sea salt and black pepper, to taste

Optional:

- 1 cup full-fat yogurt or sour cream (230 g/ 8.1 oz)

Instructions

1. Put the turkey in a bowl and add the almond flour, egg, crushed garlic, chile pepper, Dijon mustard, lemon juice, parsley, basil, salt, and black pepper. Add one finely-sliced spring onion and leave the other for garnish.
2. Mix all the ingredients until well combined and then use your hands to form small patties (about 43 g/ 1.5 oz per patty).
3. Heat the ghee in a griddle or regular pan and add the patties when hot. Don't turn the patties too soon or they will stick to the pan.

4. Cook the patties on each side until browned, working in batches and placing on a plate one at a time as they get cooked. Set aside.

5. Meanwhile, prepare the cucumber salsa. Wash the cucumber and grate into a bowl. Wash and finely chop the jalapeño pepper. Add all the remaining ingredients, including the yogurt or sour cream, if using, and mix until well combined. Serve with the turkey patties.

6. The patties can be stored in the fridge for up to 4 days. The cucumber salsa can be stored for up to a day but is best served fresh.

Prep Time: 15 Minutes

Cook Time: 20 Minutes

Servings: 4

Ingredients

- 250 g green cabbage, shredded (8.8. oz)
- 1 medium carrot, grated (60 g/ 2.1 oz)
- 100 g white mushrooms, sliced (3.5 oz)
- 3 tbsp virgin avocado oil or ghee (45 ml)
- 2 cloves garlic, minced
- 500 g ground pork (1.1 lb) - I used 5% fat
- 2 tbsp coconut aminos or tamari sauce (30 ml)
- 1 tbsp oyster sauce or fish sauce (15 ml)
- 2 tbsp apple cider vinegar (30 ml)
- 2 tbsp unsweetened tomato paste (30 ml)
- 1 tbsp Erythritol or Swerve (10 g/ 0.4 oz)
- 2 cups bean sprouts (200 g/ 7.1 oz)
- 2 medium spring onions, sliced (30 g/ 1.1 oz)
- 4 tbsp extra virgin olive oil (60 ml/ 2 fl oz)

Instructions

1. Finely slice the cabbage and grate the carrot using large holes on your grater. Slice the mushrooms.Keto Spring Roll in a Bowl

2. Place minced garlic in a skillet greased with avocado oil (or ghee). Cook for a minute until fragrant.

3. Add ground pork (I used 5% ground pork). Use a spatula to break into pieces. Cook for a minute or two, and then add the coconut aminos, oyster sauce (or use fish sauce), vinegar, tomato paste, and Erythritol.

4. Cook on medium-high for 3 to 4 minutes until browned. Add the sliced mushrooms and cook for about 3 to 5 minutes.Keto Spring Roll in a Bowl

5. Add the shredded cabbage, carrot and bean sprouts. At first this will seem like a lot but the cabbage will cook down. Using tongs, toss while cooking.

6. Cook for 6 to 8 minutes or until the cabbage is wilted and crisp tender. Take off the heat and stir in the olive oil. Optionally, season with salt and pepper to taste.Keto Spring Roll in a Bowl

7. To serve, sprinkle with spring onion. To store, let it cool down and refrigerate for up to 4 days. Reheat before serving. You can stir in the spring onion before placing in the fridge or add it just before serving.

Prep Time: 15 Minutes

Cook Time: 25 Minutes

Servings: 4

Ingredients

- 8 ounces whole-grain macaroni elbows
- 1 head of broccoli, florets cut into small bites (about 1 ½ to 2 cups), optional
- 1 ½ tablespoons avocado oil or extra-virgin olive oil
- 1 small yellow onion, chopped (about 1 ½ cups)
- 1 cup peeled and grated russet potato (4 ounces, about 1 small or ½ medium potato), preferably organic
- 3 cloves garlic, pressed or minced
- ½ teaspoon garlic powder
- ½ teaspoon onion powder
- ½ teaspoon dry mustard powder
- ½ teaspoon fine sea salt, more to taste
- Small pinch of Frontier Co-op red pepper flakes
- ⅔ cup raw cashews
- 1 cup water, more as necessary
- ¼ cup Frontier Co-op nutritional yeast

- 2 to 3 teaspoons apple cider vinegar or distilled white vinegar, to taste

Instructions

1. Bring a large pot of salted water to boil for the pasta. Cook according to package directions. If using broccoli, stir it into the pot when just 2 to 3 more minutes remain. Drain, and transfer the contents to a large serving bowl.

2. Meanwhile, in a medium-to-large saucepan, warm the oil over medium heat. Add the onion and a pinch of salt and cook, stirring often, until the onion is tender and turning translucent, about 5 minutes.

3. Add the grated potato, garlic, garlic powder, onion powder, mustard powder, salt and red pepper flakes. Stir to combine, and cook, stirring constantly, for about 1 minute to enhance their flavors.

4. Add the cashews and water, and stir to combine. Let the mixture come to a simmer. Continue simmering, stirring frequently and reducing heat as necessary to avoid a rapid boil, until the potatoes are completely tender and cooked through, about 5 to 8 minutes.

5. Carefully pour the mixture into a blender. Add the nutritional yeast and 2 teaspoons vinegar. Blend until the mixture is completely smooth, about 2 minutes, stopping to scrape down the sides if necessary. If the mixture won't blend easily or if you would prefer a thinner consistency, add water in ¼ cup increments, blending after each one.

6. Taste, and blend in additional salt until the sauce is utterly irresistible (I typically add at least another ½ teaspoon). If it needs a little more zip, add the remaining teaspoon of vinegar. Blend again.

7. Pour the sauce into the bowl of pasta. Stir until well combined, and serve immediately. Leftovers keep well, chilled and covered, for 3 to 4 days. Gentle reheat, adding a tiny splash of water if necessary to loosen up the sauce.

Prep Time: 20 Minutes

Cook Time: 35 Minutes

Servings: 4

Ingredients

- 2 tablespoons olive oil
- 1 tablespoon finely chopped fresh sage
- 2 pound butternut or kabocha squash, peeled, seeded, and cut into small ½-inch pieces (about 3 cups)
- 1 medium yellow onion, chopped
- 2 garlic cloves, pressed or chopped
- ⅛ teaspoon red pepper flakes (up to ¼ teaspoon for spicier pasta sauce)
- Salt
- Freshly ground black pepper
- 2 cups vegetable broth
- 12 ounces whole grain linguine or fettucine
- Optional additional garnishes: shaved Parmesan or Pecorino and/or smoked salt

Instructions

1. Warm the oil in a large skillet over medium heat. Once the oil is shimmering, add the sage and toss to coat. Let the sage get crispy before transferring it to a small bowl. Sprinkle it lightly with salt and set the bowl aside.

2. Add the squash, onion, garlic and red pepper flakes to the skillet. Season with salt and pepper. Cook, stirring occasionally, until the onion is translucent, about 8 to 10 minutes. Add the broth. Bring the mixture to a boil, then reduce the heat and simmer until the squash is soft and the liquid is reduced by half, about 15 to 20 minutes.

3. In the meantime, bring a large pot of salted water to a boil and cook the pasta until al dente according to package directions, stirring occasionally. Reserve 1 cup of the pasta cooking water before draining.

4. Once the squash mixture is done cooking, remove it from the heat and let it cool slightly. Transfer the contents of the pan to a blender, but keep the skillet handy. Purée the mixture until smooth (beware of hot steam escaping from the top of the blender), then season with salt and pepper until the flavors sing.

5. In the reserved skillet, combine the pasta, squash purée and ¼ cup cooking liquid. Cook over medium heat, tossing and adding more pasta cooking water as needed, until the sauce coats the pasta, about 2 minutes. Season with more salt and pepper if necessary.

6. Serve the pasta in individual bowls topped with fried sage, more black pepper and shaved Parmesan/Pecorino and/or smoked salt, if desired.

Prep Time: 10 Minutes

Cook Time: 50 Minutes

Servings: 4

Ingredients

Roasted spaghetti squash:

- 2 medium spaghetti squash (about 2 pounds each), halved and seeds removed
- 2 tablespoons olive oil
- Salt and freshly ground black pepper
- Cabbage and black bean slaw
- 2 cups purple cabbage, thinly sliced and roughly chopped into 2-inch long pieces
- 1 can (15 ounces) black beans, rinsed and drained
- 1 red bell pepper, chopped
- ⅓ cup chopped green onions, both green and white parts
- ⅓ cup chopped fresh cilantro
- 2 to 3 tablespoons fresh lime juice, to taste
- 1 teaspoon olive oil

- ¼ teaspoon salt
- Avocado salsa verde
- ¾ cup mild salsa verde, either homemade or store-bought
- 1 ripe avocado, diced
- ⅓ cup fresh cilantro (a few stems are ok)
- 1 tablespoon fresh lime juice
- 1 medium garlic clove, roughly chopped

Optional garnishes:

- chopped fresh cilantro, crumbled feta and/or seasoned toasted pepitas

Instructions

1. To roast the spaghetti squash: Preheat the oven to 400 degrees Fahrenheit and line a large baking sheet with parchment paper for easy clean-up. On the baking sheet, drizzle the halved spaghetti squash with olive oil. Rub the olive oil all over each of the halves, adding more if necessary.

2. Sprinkle the insides of the squash with freshly ground black pepper and salt. Turn them over so the insides

are facing down. Roast for 40 to 60 minutes, until the flesh is easily pierced through with a fork.

3. Meanwhile, to assemble the slaw: In a medium mixing bowl, combine the cabbage, black beans, bell pepper, green onion, cilantro, lime juice, olive oil and salt. Toss to combine and set aside to marinate.

4. To make the salsa verde: In the bowl of a blender or food processor, combine the avocado, salsa verde, cilantro, lime juice and garlic. Blend until smooth, pausing to scrape down the sides as necessary.

5. To assemble, first use a fork to separate and fluff up the flesh of the spaghetti squash. Then divide the slaw into each of the spaghetti squash "bowls," and add a big dollop of avocado salsa verde. Finish the bowls with another sprinkle of pepper, cilantro and optional crumbled feta or pepitas.

Prep Time: 20 Minutes

Cook Time: 45 Minutes

Servings: 4

Ingredients

Green rice:

- 3 tablespoons extra-virgin olive oil
- 1 ½ cups long grain brown rice
- 3 cups vegetable broth
- 1 ½ cup baby spinach, lightly packed
- ½ cup cilantro (mostly leaves, stems are ok), lightly packed
- 1 jalapeño or serrano pepper, seeded, membranes removed and roughly chopped
- 1 medium shallot, peeled and roughly chopped
- 1 garlic clove, peeled, roughly chopped
- ¼ teaspoon salt, more to taste

Sweet potatoes:

- 2 pounds sweet potatoes (3 to 4 medium sweet potatoes), peeled and sliced into 1-inch chunks

- 2 tablespoons olive oil
- ½ teaspoon smoked paprika
- ¼ teaspoon sea salt
- Seasoned black beans
- 2 cans (14 ounces each) black beans or 3 cups cooked black beans, with their cooking liquid
- 2 teaspoons ground cumin
- ½ teaspoon chili powder
- 1 teaspoon sherry vinegar or lime juice
- Sea salt and freshly ground black pepper, to taste

Additional garnishes:

- ¼ cup pepitas (green pumpkin seeds)
- ¼ teaspoon olive oil
- 1 avocado, pitted and sliced
- Jarred mild salsa verde
- Chopped cilantro
- Crumbled feta (optional, not vegan)

Instructions

1. Preheat oven to 425 degrees Fahrenheit. Line one large, rimmed baking sheet and one smaller sheet with parchment paper. Place the spinach, cilantro, jalapeño, shallot, garlic, salt and ½ cup of the

vegetable broth in a food processor or blender. Blend until smooth.

2. Heat the oil in a heavy-bottomed pot over medium heat until shimmering. Add the rice and stir to coat. Spread the rice in an even layer on the bottom of the pot and let the rice lightly brown. This happens quickly! When the rice starts to brown, stir it and spread it out in an even layer again so that more of the rice browns.

3. When most of the rice has lightly browned, scrape the green purée into the rice. Stir until the rice is evenly coated with green purée and continue to cook, stirring constantly, for a minute. Add the rest of the vegetable broth to the pot. Bring to a boil, then reduce the heat to a low simmer and cover the pot. Cook the rice on a very low simmer until tender, 35 to 40 minutes.

4. While the rice cooks, toss the sweet potatoes in the olive oil, smoked paprika and salt until the sweet potatoes are evenly coated in oil. Arrange in a single layer on your prepared baking sheet. Bake for 35 to 40 minutes, tossing halfway, until the sweet potatoes are tender and caramelizing at the edges.

5. Meanwhile, transfer the beans and their cooking liquid (don't drain the beans) to a medium pot. Stir in

the cumin and chili powder and warm over medium heat. Once the beans are simmering, cover the beans and reduce heat to maintain a very gentle simmer until you're ready to serve.

6. Once the rice is done cooking, remove the pot from heat. Uncover the pot and place a clean tea towel over the pot, then recover. The towel will help absorb excess liquid as the rice continues to cook in its own steam. (If you don't have a clean towel, you can skip this step, just cover normally.) Let sit for 10 minutes.

7. Once the sweet potatoes are done cooking, toss the pepitas with ¼ teaspoon olive oil and a sprinkle of salt on the small baking sheet. Toast the seeds in the oven for 4 to 5 minutes, until they're turning lightly golden and making little popping noises. Set aside to cool.

8. Fluff the rice with a fork and season with salt if necessary. Remove beans from heat, stir in the vinegar and season to taste with salt and pepper.

9. Assemble your bowls: First add green rice, then use a slotted spoon or fork to transfer beans to the bowls. Top with sweet potatoes and add a few slices of avocado to each bowl. Sprinkle with toasted pepitas

and cilantro and optional feta. Serve with salsa verde
on the side.

Prep Time: 30 Minutes

Cook Time: 30 Minutes

Servings: 4

Ingredients

Rice and veggies:

- 1 ¼ cups short-grain brown rice or long-grain brown rice, rinsed
- 1 ½ cups frozen shelled edamame, preferably organic
- 1 ½ cups trimmed and roughly chopped snap peas or snow peas, or thinly sliced broccoli florets
- 1 to 2 tablespoons reduced-sodium tamari or soy sauce, to taste
- 4 cups chopped red cabbage or spinach or romaine lettuce or kale (ribs removed)
- 2 ripe avocados, halved, pitted and thinly sliced into long strips (wait to slice just before serving, see details in step 5)

Essential garnishes:

- 1 small cucumber, very thinly sliced

- Carrot ginger dressing
- Thinly sliced green onion (about ½ small bunch)
- Lime wedges
- Toasted sesame oil, for drizzling
- Sesame seeds
- Flaky sea salt

Instructions

1. Bring a large pot of water to boil (ideally about 4 quarts water). Once the water is boiling, add the rice and continue boiling for 25 minutes. Add the edamame and cook for 3 more minutes (it's ok if the water doesn't reach a rapid boil again). Then add the snap peas and cook for 2 more minutes.

2. Drain well, and return the rice and veggies to the pot. Season to taste with 1 to 2 tablespoons of tamari or soy sauce, and stir to combine.

3. Divide the rice/veggie mixture and raw veggies into 4 bowls. Arrange cucumber slices along the edge of the bowl (see photos). Drizzle lightly with carrot ginger dressing and top with sliced green onion. Place a lime wedge or 2 in each bowl.

4. When you're ready to serve, divide the avocado into the bowls. Lightly drizzle sesame oil over the avocado, followed by a generous sprinkle of sesame seeds and flaky sea salt. Serve promptly.

5. If you intend to have leftovers, wait to complete step 4 just before serving (otherwise the avocado will brown too soon). Leftover bowls keep well (avocado excluded) for 4 to 5 days in the refrigerator.

Prep Time: 20 Minutes

Cook Time: 10 Minutes

Servings: 4

Ingredients

- ilantro-pepita pesto
- ⅓ cup raw pepitas (pumpkin seeds)
- 1 cup packed cilantro (mostly leaves, about 2 bunches' worth)
- 2 teaspoons seeded and roughly chopped jalapeño
- 2 cloves garlic, roughly chopped
- 1 lime, juiced
- ½ teaspoon fine-grain sea salt
- ⅓ cup extra virgin olive oil
- Pasta and squash ribbons
- 8 ounces (½ pound) whole grain fettuccine or linguine
- 2 small zucchini
- 1 yellow squash

Instructions

1. Lightly toast the pepitas in a small pan over medium-low heat for a few minutes, tossing frequently, until fragrant. Transfer the pepitas to a bowl to cool a bit.

2. Remove any discolored skin from the squash with a paring knife. Use a julienne peeler (or regular peeler) to slice the squash lengthwise, one side at a time (stop once you get to the seeded part, then turn the squash to work on the next side).

3. Bring a large pot of salted water to a boil, and cook fettuccine until al dente, according to the package's instructions. Drain and set aside.

4. In a food processor, combine the cilantro, jalapeño, garlic, lime juice, salt and cooled pepitas. While running the food processor, drizzle in the olive oil. Stop processing once the pesto is well blended.

5. Toss the cooked pasta and ribboned squash with the pesto and serve.

Prep Time: 20 Minutes

Cook Time: 20 Minutes

Servings: 4

Ingredients

Pasta and zucchini noodles:

- 8 ounces whole grain spaghetti
- 1 large zucchini

Pesto

- ⅔ cup walnuts
- 2 pints (4 cups) cherry or grape tomatoes
- 2 tablespoons olive oil, plus more for drizzling
- ¼ cup oil-packed sun-dried tomatoes, rinsed and drained
- 2 garlic cloves, roughly chopped
- ½ teaspoon finely grated lemon zest
- 1 to 2 tablespoons lemon juice
- ¼ teaspoon red pepper flakes
- ¼ teaspoon salt, to taste
- Freshly ground black pepper, to taste

Garnishes

- ½ cup lightly packed basil leaves, larger leaves torn into small pieces
- Freshly grated Parmesan cheese or vegan Parmesan, for serving (both optional)
- Olive oil, for drizzling

Instructions

1. Bring a large pot of salted water to boil for the spaghetti. Cook the pasta until al dente, according to package directions. Drain and transfer to a large serving bowl. Spiralize the zucchini with a spiralizer (here's how), or turn the zucchini into noodles with a julienne peeler, or grate the zucchini the long way on a large box grater.
2. Toast the walnuts: In a medium skillet over medium heat, cook the walnuts, stirring occasionally, until they smell nice and fragrant, about 7 minutes. Set aside to cool.
3. Cook the cherry tomatoes: In a large saucepan over medium-high heat, combine the cherry tomatoes, olive oil and a pinch of salt. Cover the pot and cook, stirring occasionally, until the tomatoes have burst

open and they are cooking in their own juices, about 7 to 8 minutes. Set aside.

4. In a food processor, combine the walnuts, half of the cooked tomatoes, sun-dried tomatoes, garlic, lemon zest, 1 tablespoon lemon juice, red pepper flakes, ¼ teaspoon salt and several twists of freshly ground black pepper. Blend until the mixture is pretty smooth, then season to taste with additional lemon juice, salt and/or pepper until the flavors really sing (if that doesn't do the trick, add some more sun-dried tomatoes). Blend again.

5. Pour the pesto over the spaghetti and toss to combine. If you'll be consuming this dish in one sitting, go ahead and toss in all of the zucchini noodles now, too. (If you plan on having leftovers, store the zucchini noodles separately from the rest, as they leach water when they're exposed to salt—I just pile the noodles on top of my individual bowls and wait to stir them in when I'm ready to eat. Hope that makes sense.)

6. Pour the rest of the cherry tomatoes on top of the dish, and sprinkle the basil over them. Toss gently, and divide the mixture into bowls. Top individual bowls with Parmesan or nutritional yeast, if you'd like, and a light drizzle of olive oil. Serve immediately.

www.ingramcontent.com/pod-product-compliance
Lightning Source LLC
Chambersburg PA
CBHW070955250726
48663CB00002B/240